COPD DIET COOKBOOK:

FOR NEWLY DIAGNOSED

Complete Beginner Procedures On Foods, Meal Plan Recipes + Healthy Lifestyle Tips To Manage, Strive, And Live Well With Chronic Obstructive Pulmonary Disease

DR. EMMY BROOKS

ABOUT THIS BOOK

In the enlightening pages of the "COPD Diet Cookbook," readers embark on a transformative journey towards better respiratory health through the lens of nutrition. The book's introduction sets the stage by providing a comprehensive overview of Chronic Obstructive Pulmonary Disease (COPD) and delves into the pivotal role a COPD-friendly diet plays in supporting respiratory well-being. Aiming to be a beacon of guidance, this cookbook seamlessly weaves together the intricate relationship between COPD and nutrition.

Exploring the synergy between COPD and nutrition, the book's initial chapters unravel the impact of the disease on dietary needs, elucidating the pivotal role that a well-crafted diet can play in managing symptoms and enhancing overall quality of life. It goes beyond theory, empowering readers with practical advice on building a COPD-friendly pantry, stocking up on essential ingredients, and mastering the art of smart grocery shopping and meal planning.

The heart of the book lies in its delectable recipes thoughtfully designed to cater to respiratory health. From quick and nutrient-packed breakfasts to energizing lunches and flavorful dinners, each dish is a harmonious blend of taste and nutritional efficacy. Snack options for on-the-go moments and hydration strategies for COPD further round out the culinary adventure, ensuring a comprehensive approach to sustaining respiratory wellness.

Delving into the nitty-gritty, the cookbook equips readers with cooking techniques tailored for respiratory wellness, advocating for the best methods to preserve nutrients and minimize irritants during food preparation. Practical kitchen hacks and time-saving tips for efficient meal preparation seamlessly integrate into the narrative, offering a helping hand in creating a COPD-friendly cooking environment.

Beyond the kitchen, the book extends its guidance to the challenges of dining out, offering strategies for navigating restaurant menus and communicating dietary needs effectively. It doesn't stop there; it addresses the broader spectrum of maintaining a COPD-friendly lifestyle, tackling common challenges, and offering long-term strategies for seamless integration into daily life.

In this engaging and uplifting tone, the "COPD Diet Cookbook" becomes more than a collection of recipes; it transforms into a trusted companion on the journey to better respiratory health. Through its pages, readers find not only a guide to nourishing meals but also a source of encouragement, motivation, and celebration for every step taken towards a healthier, COPD-friendly lifestyle.

DISCLAIMER

This book's content is solely intended for general informative purposes. About the availability, applicability, correctness, completeness, and trustworthiness of the data or recipes in this book, the author provides no guarantees of any sort, either stated or implied. You bear full responsibility for any reliance you may have on such material.

The advice, diagnosis, or treatment provided by a qualified medical expert is not to be replaced by this cookbook. When in doubt about a medical problem, never hesitate to consult your doctor or another trained healthcare professional. Never ignore medical advice from professionals or put off getting it because of something you've read in this book.

At the time of publishing, the author of this book has taken reasonable steps to guarantee that the information is correct and current. He does not, however, guarantee that the data will be error-free or that it will satisfy any certain performance or quality standards.

Any negative repercussions that may arise from using or applying the material in this book are not the responsibility of the author, publisher, or distributor.

In this book, references or mentions of individuals, products, websites, organizations, or other names are for informational purposes only and do not imply endorsement or affiliation with the author. The author has no control over the nature, content, and availability of referenced or mentioned entities. Any reliance on such information is at the reader's own risk.

The inclusion of any references does not necessarily imply a recommendation or endorse the views expressed within them. The author or publisher shall not be liable for any loss or damage arising out of or in connection with, the use of this book.

By reading and using the information in this book, you agree to the terms of this disclaimer. If you do not agree with these terms, please refrain from using this book.

INTRODUCTION

OVERVIEW of COPD (Chronic Obstructive Pulmonary Disease)

The term "chronic obstructive pulmonary disease" (COPD) refers to a group of lung disorders, including emphysema and chronic bronchitis, that are common and progressing. It is typified by restricted airflow, which can cause coughing, breathing problems, and a higher risk of respiratory infections. People with COPD frequently have a lower quality of life because of restrictions on their everyday activities and general health.

Anyone living with COPD must have a thorough understanding of the illness to appropriately manage their symptoms. The main cause of the illness is extended exposure to irritants such as air pollution, cigarette smoke, and work-related dangers. These conditions deteriorate the lungs over time and impair their capacity to operate at their best, leading to ongoing breathing difficulties.

We will explore the intricacies of COPD in this cookbook, offering crucial details regarding its causes, manifestations, and available treatments. People with COPD are more equipped to make decisions about their health and modify their lifestyles in ways that will improve their respiratory health.

The Value of a Diet Appropriate for COPD

To control COPD symptoms and enhance general respiratory health, diet is essential. A thoughtfully planned diet for people with COPD can help with several things, including supplying vital nutrients, keeping weight in check, and reducing the chance of flare-ups. Because of symptoms including weariness, dyspnea, and decreased appetite, people with COPD frequently struggle to eat healthily.

The significance of a well-balanced diet customized to fulfill the specific requirements of people with COPD is emphasized in this cookbook. Foods high in nutrients can improve energy levels, strengthen respiratory muscles, and build the immune system. Furthermore, keeping a healthy weight is essential for controlling COPD since being overweight puts stress on the respiratory system and makes it more difficult for people to breathe.

We'll look at doable and tasty dishes that not only meet the dietary needs of people with COPD but also take into account any preparation, cooking, and consuming difficulties they could encounter. People with COPD can improve their overall health and respiratory health by taking proactive measures to recognize the importance of a diet that is friendly to their condition.

How The Nutrition In This Recipe Is Intended To Enhance Respiratory Health

This cookbook is intended to serve as a thorough reference for people with COPD as they pursue improved lung health via diet. It's more than just a cookbook; it offers insightful information about the nutrients that are essential for COPD management. Every recipe is painstakingly created using components high in antioxidants, vitamins, and minerals that are especially beneficial to respiratory health.

The handbook provides beginners with detailed directions that guarantee cooking ease without compromising taste or nutrition. We are aware of the particular issues that people with COPD may encounter, such as low energy and sometimes challenging meal preparation. As a result, the recipes are designed to be both nourishing and simple to follow, so anyone with different levels of culinary skill can use them.

Additionally, the cookbook delves into the idea of meal planning, enabling people to design a balanced, COPD-friendly diet that satisfies their dietary requirements. The cookbook attempts to make the process fun and sustainable by combining a range of flavors and ingredients, inspiring people to make a long-term commitment to lung health through mindful eating.

In the sections that follow, we'll go into more detail on particular recipes, dietary recommendations, and helpful hints to help both inexperienced and seasoned cooks enjoy the process of transitioning to a COPD-friendly diet.

Advice For Readers Seeking To Improve Their Diet-Based Respiratory Health:

Setting out on a nutritional path to improve respiratory health can be enjoyable and demanding at the same time. As readers immerse themselves in the COPD Diet Cookbook, it is critical to recognize the importance of their dedication to enhancing their health. On this route, a good outlook and tenacity are vital allies.

Above all, readers should be proud of themselves for being proactive in controlling their COPD symptoms with food choices. It's an arduous trip, and each little victory is celebrated along the way. Embracing the potential of nutrient-dense meals is essential for mental and emotional wellness in addition to physical health.

It is essential to set reasonable goals. Making small, lasting changes over time can be more beneficial than trying for big, quick fixes. With the help of the cookbook, adopting COPD-friendly foods into daily life may be made easy and pleasurable. Establishing realistic goals, like trying out one new meal every week, makes improvement more manageable and long-lasting.

Another important part of this process is asking for help. Having a network of supporters, whether they be family members, friends, or medical professionals, can be very beneficial. Communicate your objectives, difficulties, and successes to those in your vicinity. This promotes a sense of community in addition to accountability.

The trip can become a culinary adventure by experimenting with flavors and recipes. The cookbook makes sure that readers can find dishes that fit their dietary requirements and preferences by providing a wide range of tasty and nutritious options. It can be exciting to try new foods and flavors, transforming a required dietary change into a delightful culinary adventure.

Finally, persistence is essential. Nutritional management of COPD is an ongoing effort, and setbacks are possible. It's critical to see every day as a fresh chance to make better decisions. Long-term success in using nutrition to manage COPD symptoms will depend on gaining knowledge from experiences, maintaining resilience, and making necessary dietary adjustments. Everybody's journey is different, but with commitment and help from the COPD Diet Cookbook, readers can achieve the best possible respiratory health and a higher standard of living.

CHAPTER ONE

KNOWLEDGE OF NUTRITION AND COPD

A Synopsis of COPD and How It Affects Nutrition

Emphysema and chronic bronchitis are two ailments that are included in the progressive lung disease known as chronic obstructive pulmonary disease, or COPD. It is typified by chronic respiratory discomfort, restricted airflow, and airway inflammation. A person's nutritional health can be significantly impacted by COPD because of the higher energy costs linked to respiratory problems and decreased lung function.

The narrowing of the airways caused by COPD makes it harder for air to enter and exit the lungs. Individuals may thus suffer from exhaustion, a persistent cough, and shortness of breath. These symptoms might worsen the nutritional difficulties that people with COPD have by causing a decrease in appetite and weight loss.

Sustaining a healthy diet is essential for successful COPD management. Breathing becomes more difficult when one's respiratory muscles are weakened due to poor nutritional status. Malnutrition can also weaken the immune system, which raises the possibility of infections and worsening. It is crucial to comprehend the connection between nutrition and COPD to create a diet that promotes general health and well-being.

The Dietary Requirements of People with COPD

To meet the nutritional demands of people with COPD, particular issues with energy expenditure, weight maintenance, and nutrient intake must be resolved. For those with COPD, consuming enough calories is essential to meet their increased energy needs due to breathing difficulties. However, due to things like weariness, dyspnea (shortness of breath), and decreased appetite, this can be difficult to achieve.

To overcome these obstacles, people with COPD should concentrate on eating nutrient-dense foods that include vital vitamins and minerals without adding too many calories. Lean protein sources—like fish, poultry, tofu, and legumes—are crucial for preserving respiratory health and muscle mass. Eating a wide range of vibrant fruits and vegetables guarantees a plentiful supply of antioxidants, which can aid in the reduction of inflammation and promote the general health of the lungs.

People with COPD must keep a close eye on their weight and collaborate with medical providers to create a customized eating plan. Individual dietary preferences, dietary limitations, and the unique requirements of managing COPD should all be considered in this strategy. Additionally, it's critical to drink enough water because dehydration can worsen respiratory symptoms and increase fatigue.

Diet's Function in Controlling Symptoms and Enhancing Life Quality

An intelligently designed and balanced diet is essential for controlling COPD symptoms and enhancing general quality of life. People with COPD can optimize their nutritional intake to promote respiratory function and improve their overall well-being by focusing on particular dietary principles.

First of all, controlling portion sizes is crucial to avoiding overeating because being overweight can aggravate respiratory conditions by straining the respiratory muscles. Throughout the day, eating smaller, more frequent meals can assist control energy levels without overtaxing the digestive system.

For people with COPD, selecting foods that are simple to chew and swallow is essential because breathing problems can make eating difficult. Foods that are soft, moist, and cooked through are the best; additionally, adding sauces, gravies, or healthy fats to meals can improve their flavor and moisture content.

Controlling sodium consumption is also important because too much salt can exacerbate respiratory symptoms and lead to fluid retention. Limiting the consumption of packaged and processed foods and choosing fresh, unprocessed foods can help manage salt intake.

The anti-inflammatory properties of omega-3 fatty acids from foods like walnuts, flaxseeds, and fatty fish may help to lessen airway inflammation. Furthermore, sustaining respiratory function and avoiding dehydration depends on maintaining a healthy level of fluid consumption, ideally water.

Working along with medical specialists, such as pulmonologists and dietitians, is crucial for customizing dietary advice to each patient's requirements and tracking how dietary modifications affect COPD control. People with COPD can improve their nutritional status, reduce symptoms, and eventually live better by using a customized, well-balanced diet.

CHAPTER TWO

CONSTRUCTING A COPD-COMPATIBLE PANTRY
Crucial Elements in a Diet Suitable for People with COPD:

It is important to concentrate on ingredients that support lung health, offer vital nutrients, and are simple to prepare when building a pantry that is COPD-friendly. Start with lean proteins, such as fish, lentils, and skinless chicken. In addition to being high in amino acids, these protein sources are low in saturated fats, which is advantageous for those with COPD. Choose whole grains such as quinoa, brown rice, and oats; they are easy on the stomach and include a decent amount of fiber and other important minerals.

Your COPD-friendly pantry should be centered around fresh fruits and vegetables. Rich in vitamins, minerals, and antioxidants, they support immune system performance as well as general health.

Colorful foods that offer a variety of health benefits include cruciferous vegetables, citrus fruits, berries, and leafy greens. But be aware of certain triggers; some people with COPD might have to stay away from certain raw veggies that can make them bloated or gassy.

Nuts, avocados, and olive oil are good sources of healthy fats that are essential for preserving lung health. Omega-3 fatty acids, which are abundant in these fats and have anti-inflammatory qualities, may help lessen COPD symptoms.

Adding low-fat dairy or dairy substitutes also guarantees a sufficient intake of calcium and vitamin D, which are essential for healthy bones.

Herbs and spices are great options for seasoning food without resorting to too much salt. To control blood pressure and fluid retention, many COPD patients must keep an eye on their sodium intake. Herbs such as rosemary, thyme, and basil can enhance flavor without sacrificing nutrition.

Purchasing Nutritious Staples in Bulk:

Choosing nutrient-dense staples that may serve as the basis for well-balanced meals is the first step in creating a pantry that is COPD-friendly. Your pantry should be stocked with whole grains since they are a dependable source of carbs that will provide you with energy for the entire day. In addition to providing complex carbs, foods like brown rice and quinoa also include fiber, which is good for the digestive system.

Make certain that a range of lean proteins is easily accessible. Tuna, lentils, and canned beans are easy and varied sources of protein. To limit salt intake, choose canned foods with minimal sodium content. Another great source of protein is eggs, which can be used in a variety of recipes and supply the vital amino acids needed to keep muscles healthy.

Keep a wide variety of fresh and frozen fruits and veggies on hand. While frozen choices are more convenient and have a longer shelf life, fresh food gives meals more brightness. Broccoli, carrots, spinach, and berries are all great options because they include a variety of vitamins and minerals.

Add some healthy fats to your cupboard to boost the nutritional value and taste. Nuts, seeds, and olive oil are excellent providers of mono- and polyunsaturated fats that support lung and heart function. Nut butter, like peanut or almond butter, can be added to smoothies to increase their nutritional value or spread on whole-grain toast.

Remember to consume dairy products or dairy substitutes to meet your needs for calcium and vitamin D. Cheese, Greek yogurt, and fortified almond milk are adaptable choices that may be included in a variety of dishes to guarantee a balanced diet.

Advice for Conscientious Food Buying and Meal Planning:

Planning meals and grocery shopping ahead of time is crucial to keeping a diet that is COPD-friendly. Make a thorough shopping list first, taking inspiration from your food plan. Using this list will not only keep you organized but also stop you from making impulsive purchases that might not be in line with your diet plans.

Pay attention to the periphery of the grocery store when browsing the aisles as this is where fresh vegetables, lean proteins, and dairy are usually found. This tactic reduces exposure to packaged and processed foods high in harmful fats and sodium while promoting healthier choices.

When feasible, try to buy in bulk, especially for non-perishables like nuts, beans, and whole grains. Purchasing in bulk guarantees a steady supply of necessary components in your pantry while also saving money.

Choose whole, fresh foods over processed and prepackaged ones. Less additives and greater nutritional value are found in fresh fruits, vegetables, and lean proteins. When choosing packaged foods, check the labels for sodium levels and, if possible, choose low-sodium or no-added-salt options.

Make meal plans that are both reasonable in terms of preparation time and rich in nutrients. Maintaining a healthy eating regimen is made easier and stress is reduced by using simple recipes that require few steps. To speed up the cooking process on hectic days, think about bulk cooking or prepping parts of meals.

To sum up, careful meal planning and strategic food buying are essential elements of a successful COPD-friendly diet. A well-balanced and respiratory-friendly pantry can be created by people by emphasizing nutrient-dense staples, choosing a range of fresh and whole foods, and developing efficient shopping routines. These actions will promote their overall health and well-being.

CHAPTER THREE

EASY AND PACKED WITH NUTRIENTS BREAKFASTS
Breakfast Ideas Developed with Respiratory Health in Mind

1. Fresh Berries and Nuts with Oatmeal:

A nutritious cup of oats is a great way to start the day for those on a diet that is COPD-friendly. Soluble fiber, which improves digestion and keeps blood sugar levels steady, is abundant in oats. After bringing milk or water to a boil, add the rolled oats. Cook until the oats are creamy in consistency.

Throw in a handful of fresh berries, such as strawberries or blueberries, to increase the nutritious content. Antioxidants, which are abundant in these fruits, support respiratory health in general. For extra protein and good fats, sprinkle some nuts, such as walnuts or almonds, on top of your porridge.

Additionally, nuts offer vital minerals that support lung function, such as vitamin E and magnesium.

2. Toast with avocado and smoked salmon:

Avocado toast with smoked salmon is a delicious and filling choice for a breakfast that is suitable for those with COPD. Avocados are rich in potassium and heart-healthy monounsaturated fats, which are good for those with respiratory disorders. Mash a ripe avocado and evenly distribute it over whole-grain toast to prepare.

Add slices of smoked salmon next; salmon is a great source of omega-3 fatty acids, which are believed to have anti-inflammatory effects. These good fats can improve respiratory health by helping to lessen airway irritation. Add some chia seeds to your bread as a garnish to up the omega-3s and fiber content and make your breakfast more filling and balanced.

3. Granola, fresh fruit, and Greek yogurt parfait: Greek yogurt's rich protein content and gut-healthy bacteria make it an excellent option for a COPD diet. Layer the Greek yogurt, granola, and fresh fruit to make a delectable parfait. Pour Greek yogurt into a glass or bowl to start.

Top with a layer of granola, ideally one that is high in fiber and low in sugar. Granola offers vital nutrition and long-lasting energy. Add a choice of fresh fruits, such as sliced bananas, mango, or kiwi, to the parfait; these are all high in vitamins and minerals that are essential for respiratory health. This combination guarantees the right amount of nutrients for a breakfast that is COPD-friendly in addition to providing a delicious taste.

4. Egg and Vegetable Scramble:

Try a veggie and egg scramble for a tasty and high-protein breakfast. In addition to being a great source of high-quality protein, eggs also have minerals like choline, which is good for your lungs. Start by using olive oil to sauté a variety of vibrant veggies, including tomatoes, spinach, and bell peppers.

Add the beaten eggs to the pan with the softened veggies and scramble until the eggs are cooked through. Use herbs such as chives or parsley to add flavor to the scramble without adding too much salt. This simple and quick recipe is a great option for those with COPD since it has a balanced amount of protein, vitamins, and antioxidants.

5. Blender bowl containing leafy green vegetables:

A delightful and easy approach to including nutrient-dense foods in your morning is with smoothie bowls. Blend leafy greens like spinach or kale with fruits like bananas and pineapple, along with a small amount of almond milk, to make a green smoothie bowl. The fruits give natural sweetness and extra nutrition, and the leafy greens supply vital vitamins and antioxidants.

Transfer the smoothie into a bowl and garnish with chopped almonds, chia seeds, and fresh berries, among other toppings. This breakfast choice provides a filling and revitalizing start to the day while also meeting the dietary requirements of a COPD-friendly diet.

6. Breakfast Bowl of Quinoa with Mixed Berries: A breakfast bowl full of nutrients can be made using the adaptable grain quinoa. Prepare the quinoa as directed on the package and combine it with a choice of mixed berries. Antioxidant-rich berries, such as raspberries and blackberries, are beneficial for respiratory health.

For added sweetness and crunch, drizzle some honey or maple syrup over the quinoa. You may also sprinkle chopped almonds on top for extra nutrition. With its blend of fiber, antioxidants, and complex carbohydrates, this quinoa breakfast dish is a healthy option for those on a diet that is suitable for people with COPD.

Simple to Follow Preparation Steps

The instructions for each of these nutrient-dense breakfasts are made to be easily understood by beginners, so even people who are not experienced cooks may make a satisfying breakfast. To expedite the cooking process, begin by assembling all required ingredients and tools.

For each recipe, follow the directions step-by-step; however, don't be afraid to adjust them to suit your tastes or dietary needs.

Variations to Suit Various Taste Preferences

When it comes to satisfying a range of taste preferences, adaptability is essential. Feel free to play about with the amounts of ingredients, swap out items according to dietary requirements or personal tastes, and investigate various flavor profiles. For instance, someone who likes their breakfast a little sweeter can top it off with some fruit or honey. However, people who prefer savory flavors can play around with different kinds of protein sources, herbs, and spices.

To sum up, these breakfast recipes provide a range of options for people on a COPD-friendly diet, with simple instructions and customizable versions to accommodate varying palates. Having a nutrient-rich breakfast is an easy yet powerful method to promote respiratory health and make the most of your day.

CHAPTER FOUR

ENERGIZING LUNCHES FOR RESPIRATORY SUPPORT

Lunch Options That Emphasize Respiratory Health And Energy

Rich in Nutrient Salad Bowls

A nutrient-rich salad bowl is a great lunch choice for people with COPD. Dark, leafy greens like spinach or kale, which are abundant in vital vitamins and minerals, should make up the foundation of your dish. With nutrients like vitamin C—known for its antioxidant qualities—these greens offer a strong basis for respiratory health. Incorporate an assortment of vibrant veggies such as carrots, bell peppers, and tomatoes to improve the salad's appearance and nutrient value.

Add lean proteins, like quinoa, chickpeas, or grilled chicken, to increase energy levels. Protein is essential for preserving muscular mass, which is especially critical for people with respiratory disorders. A handful of nuts or seeds can also be added for texture and beneficial fats that support overall well-being.

Seared Grain Wraps

Whole grain wraps with salmon are a great option for a meal that provides both energy and respiratory support. Complex carbs, which are found in whole grains like whole wheat, are an excellent source of energy that is released gradually throughout the day. Choosing whole grains also guarantees more fiber, which is beneficial to the health of the digestive system.

Because it is high in omega-3 fatty acids, salmon is a great option for those with COPD. Because of their anti-inflammatory qualities, omega-3s may be good for respiratory health. Instead of using too much salt, use herbs and spices to season the fish. To improve the nutritional profile and make the meal look better, add a range of vibrant veggies, such as red onions, cucumbers, and leafy greens, to the wrap.

Quinoa Stir-Fry with Veggies

Quinoa and veggie stir-fry is a quick and easy lunch alternative that's packed with nutrients. Because it contains all of the essential amino acids, quinoa is a complete protein and a great option for those with COPD. Its high fiber content promotes sustained energy throughout the day by assisting with digestion and blood sugar regulation.

Saute a variety of vibrant veggies, such as bell peppers, broccoli, and snap peas, in olive oil to make the stir-fry. Toss in the cooked quinoa and mix everything. Use seasonings like garlic, ginger, and turmeric, which have anti-inflammatory properties in addition to improving flavor. For respiratory support, this quick and simple stir-fry guarantees a pleasant and well-balanced meal.

Nutrient And Taste Balance For Filling Meals

Delicious Soups Made with COPD-Friendly Substances

Making tasty soups using ingredients that are pleasant to people with COPD is a great way to guarantee a filling and high-nutrient meal. For best results, start with a low-sodium broth foundation to avoid needless fluid retention. Select a range of vegetables, including spinach, carrots, and celery, as they are high in nutrients that are good for the respiratory system.

Think about including lean sources of protein, such as beans or shredded chicken. Herbs and spices can improve the flavor without using too much salt. Because of its anti-inflammatory qualities, turmeric is a fantastic addition to soups.

Add some nutritious grains, such as quinoa or brown rice, to the soup to make it heartier and more satisfying. This combination produces a tasty, well-balanced lunch that is ideal for those with COPD.

Avocado and Sweet Potato Bake

For respiratory support, baked sweet potatoes with avocado are a tasty and nourishing lunch choice. Beta-carotene, which is abundant in sweet potatoes and helps maintain lung health, is converted by the body into vitamin A. Sweet potatoes can have their natural sweetness enhanced and their nutrients preserved with ease by baking them.

Mash the avocado to add healthy fats and a creamy texture to the cooked sweet potato. Monounsaturated fats, which promote heart health, are abundant in avocados. For extra taste, add a splash of lime juice and a pinch of sea salt. This meal offers vital nutrients for lung health in addition to satisfying the palate.

Berries & Greek Yogurt Parfait

Berries and Greek yogurt provide a delicious and wholesome lunch option that strikes a balance between flavors and nutrients. Protein-rich Greek yogurt increases energy levels and muscle power. Choosing a basic, unsweetened variety can help you stay away from additional sugars, which can aggravate inflammation.

Arrange a mix of vibrant berries, like blueberries, raspberries, and strawberries, on top of the Greek yogurt. Antioxidants, which are abundant in berries, are essential in preventing oxidative stress in the body. Add a handful of granola or chopped nuts for extra crunch and nutrition. This parfait is a great lunch option for people with COPD since it's visually appealing and offers a pleasing blend of flavors and textures.

Adding components that are COPD-friendly to regular lunches

Select Lean Proteins

The first step in incorporating COPD-friendly ingredients into regular lunches is to select lean meats. Choose foods like tofu, fish, lentils, and skinless chicken. These proteins supply the vital amino acids required to keep muscles strong, which is important for people with respiratory disorders. Steer clear of processed and high-fat meats since they might aggravate respiratory conditions and cause inflammation.

Stress Whole Grains

A meal that is COPD-friendly should also prioritize healthy grains. Whole grains, which are high in fiber and offer a consistent flow of energy, include brown rice, quinoa, and whole wheat. Blood sugar regulation and digestion are aided by fiber, which promotes general health. To guarantee a balanced and wholesome lunch, use whole grain options for salad dressings, wraps, and sandwiches.

Make colorful vegetables a priority.

To improve the nutritional value and taste of regular lunches, add a range of vibrant veggies to your meals. Broccoli, carrots, bell peppers, leafy greens, and other vegetables are full of vitamins, minerals, and antioxidants that help maintain respiratory health. For maximum advantages to lung function, try to have a rainbow of colors on your plate to ensure a wide variety of nutrients.

Nuts and Avocados Provide Good Fats

Daily lunches must contain healthy fats for those with COPD. Nuts and avocados are great sources of monounsaturated fats, which support heart health and give food a filling texture. Nuts can be added to yogurt parfaits or mixed into salads, while avocado can be eaten on its own or added to wraps and salads. These fats improve general respiratory health in addition to making meals taste better.

Carefully Using Spices and Herbs to Season

When flavoring your food, use herbs and spices sparingly rather than adding too much salt. Herbs that enhance flavor and complexity without increasing salt content include basil, oregano, and thyme. Furthermore, anti-inflammatory spices like garlic, ginger, and turmeric are beneficial to those with COPD. Try blending various herbs and spices to find flavors that complement your taste buds and promote lung health.

Hydration with Herbal Teas and Infused Water

Make sure you stay hydrated throughout the day by selecting COPD-friendly drinks like herbal teas and flavored water. For people with respiratory disorders, maintaining adequate hydration is crucial since it promotes lung health overall and mucus production. To make a cool, tasty beverage, add slices of citrus fruit, cucumber, or mint to the water. You can drink hot or cold herbal teas, such as peppermint or chamomile, to help hydrate and support healthy breathing.

Thus, creating nutritious meals for respiratory support within the parameters of a diet-friendly to COPD requires careful component selection and careful cooking techniques. People with COPD can have enjoyable and nutritional meals by including nutrient-rich salads, whole grain wraps, aromatic soups, and balanced options like baked sweet potatoes or Greek yogurt parfaits. Incorporating lean meats, entire grains, vibrant veggies, healthy fats, and careful seasoning into daily meals guarantees a comprehensive approach to respiratory health. In addition, drinking herbal teas and infused water to stay hydrated promotes general health and supports ideal lung function. Even beginners can easily and confidently create lunches that are COPD-friendly by following these helpful guidelines.

CHAPTER FIVE

SNACKS TO IMPROVE RESPIRATORY HEALTH
Snack Selections that Promote Lung Health:

For those who have COPD, maintaining respiratory health is essential, and a vital part of controlling the illness is including snacks in the diet that promote lung function. Nutrients including vitamins, omega-3 fatty acids, and antioxidants that support respiratory health should be abundant in these snacks.

A handful of nuts, especially almonds, is a great option. Almonds are a food that is high in nutrients and a great source of antioxidants, magnesium, and vitamin E. Particularly well-known for supporting lung function and shielding cells from oxidative stress is vitamin E. Snacking on a small number of almonds can help promote respiratory health in general.

Berries are another healthy snack that is good for the lungs. Antioxidants such as flavonoids and vitamin C are abundant in berries, like strawberries and blueberries. In addition to lowering inflammation, these antioxidants shield the lungs from oxidative damage. To improve your respiratory health, try creating a cool berry smoothie or having a bowl of mixed berries as a snack.

Including foods rich in omega-3 fatty acids, such as chia or flaxseeds, can also be advantageous. Because of their anti-inflammatory qualities, omega-3 fatty acids may be able to reduce respiratory system inflammation. These seeds make a delightful and nourishing snack that promotes lung function. Sprinkle them over yogurt or blend them into a smoothie.

Realistic Actions for Beginners:

It's crucial to begin with small, doable steps for anyone new to adding lung-supportive snacks to their COPD diet. Make a list of healthy food options for your respiratory system, like almonds, berries, and seeds. Next, pick a snack that you can easily fit into your regular schedule and is easily accessible.

If you decide to go with almonds, get a tiny bag of raw or roasted almonds from your neighborhood supermarket. Stock up on these for easy and quick snacking. To make things even easier, think about portioning almonds ahead of time into tiny snack-sized containers so you always have a lung-friendly alternative on hand when hunger comes.

Choose from either fresh or frozen berries at your local grocery shop. Prepare and wash them ahead of time, then put them in the fridge in portion-sized containers. This eliminates the need for labor-intensive preparation and makes it simple to grab a nutritious snack.

Get a small jar and keep it in your cabinet for omega-3-rich seeds, such as chia or flaxseeds. It's simple to include these seeds in smoothies, yogurt, or even salad dressings. Try out several combos to discover a snack that meets your requirements for respiratory health and taste.

Snacks that are Easy to Make and Carry:

Eating a diet that is COPD-friendly doesn't have to be inconvenient. For people with COPD who are constantly on the go, many convenient and simple-to-prepare foods support lung health.

A handmade trail mix that has several components that help the lungs is one such choice. Almonds, walnuts, and pumpkin seeds can be combined to create a vitamin E, omega-3 fatty acid, and antioxidant-rich combination. For an extra flavor boost and added respiratory benefits, add some dried berries. Divide this trail mix into tiny snack packs for a quick and healthy on-the-go meal that promotes lung function.

Another easy and portable snack is a yogurt parfait with extra toppings that are good for the lungs. For added antioxidants, top the base—a plain, low-fat yogurt—with a handful of blueberries or strawberries. For added omega-3 goodness, top it with a sprinkling of flaxseeds or chia seeds.

For a hassle-free snack, you can eat anywhere, make these parfaits ahead of time, and store them in reusable containers.

Apart from low-preparation snacks, think about including pre-cut veggies paired with guacamole or hummus. In addition to being incredibly convenient, vegetables like bell pepper strips, cucumber slices, and carrot sticks also contain important vitamins and minerals. Serving them with a dip made from heart-healthy chickpeas or avocados boosts lung health and provides additional nourishment.

Realistic Actions for Beginners:

It doesn't have to be difficult to prepare portable, quick snacks for those who are often on the go, especially those who are new to using food to manage their COPD. Choose a few snacks, like trail mix, yogurt parfaits, or veggie sticks with dip, that are in line with respiratory health.

If you decide to make your trail mix, make minor purchases of the required ingredients.

Sort the portions into a bowl by measuring them out to suit your tastes. After the trail mix has been combined, divide it up into little, airtight bags or containers for easy access while traveling.

Select a yogurt variety for yogurt parfaits based on your dietary needs and taste preferences. Acquire the chosen fruits and seeds; pre-wash and chop the fruits; and store them in serving-sized containers. Just arrange the yogurt, fruits, and seeds in a carry-along container when you're ready to eat your snack.

Choose a variety of fresh veggies, such as carrots, cucumbers, and bell peppers that are simple to chop and snack on when making vegetable sticks with dip. Prepare or buy a dip, such as guacamole or hummus, and portion it into tiny jars.

Organize the veggie sticks and dip them into a travel-friendly snack container for a wholesome and convenient grab-and-go choice.

Ensuring Nutritional Value in Between Meals:

For those with COPD, preserving nutritional balance in between meals is crucial since it promotes general health and facilitates efficient COPD management. For optimum health, it is imperative to make sure that snacks have a balance of macronutrients (proteins, carbs, and fats) and micronutrients (vitamins and minerals).

Greek yogurt can help you accomplish this if you include it in your snack rotation. Greek yogurt has microorganisms that help maintain digestive health in addition to being high in protein. For extra taste and nutritional benefit, try adding a handful of almonds or a honey drizzle to a plain, low-fat Greek yogurt. This snack option promotes sustained energy between meals by ensuring a suitable balance of healthy fats and protein.

A whole grain cracker paired with lean protein, such as chicken or turkey pieces, is another nutrient-dense snack to think about. The lean protein promotes satiety and aids in maintaining muscle mass, while the whole grain crackers supply complex carbohydrates. For those with COPD who might require more protein and energy to sustain their respiratory function, this combination is perfect.

Including vitamin C-rich fruits, such as kiwis or oranges, can further improve the nutritional value in between meals. Vitamin C is well-known for boosting immune system function and having antioxidant qualities. To ensure that you always have a cool, wholesome snack on hand, keep pre-cut fruit servings in the refrigerator for convenient access.

Realistic Actions for Beginners:

Getting enough nutrition in between meals is a key component of diet-based COPD management. If you're new to this strategy, it's crucial to select snacks that fit the dietary requirements of people with respiratory disorders and are simple to prepare.

Choose a plain, low-fat Greek yogurt from your neighborhood grocery shop to begin incorporating Greek yogurt into your regimen. Get a small jar and try flavoring it with a drizzle of honey or a handful of almonds. Stock up on these items for easy, wholesome snacks in between meals.

Buying a box of whole-grain crackers and lean protein sources, like turkey or chicken slices, is an excellent choice when choosing whole-grain crackers with lean protein. To make it easy to get a healthy and delicious snack when needed, portion the protein and crackers ahead of time into snack-sized quantities.

When it comes to fruits that are high in vitamin C, pick fruits like kiwis or oranges at your next grocery store. These fruits should be cleaned, peeled, and chopped into little pieces before being kept in the refrigerator for convenient access. Keeping pre-cut fruit on hand makes it simple to grab a wholesome, immune-boosting snack in between meals.

CHAPTER SIX

SAVOURY AND PACKED WITH NUTRIENTS DINNERS

Dinner Ideas Designed with Respiratory Health in Mind

Developing dinner dishes that are specific to people with Chronic Obstructive Pulmonary Disease (COPD) means choosing products and cooking techniques that promote lung health with consideration. Including foods high in antioxidants, vitamins, and minerals with anti-inflammatory qualities is one important thing to think about. These nutrients are essential for maintaining general lung function and lowering respiratory system inflammation.

Start by incorporating your dinner preparations with an assortment of vibrant vegetables. Broccoli, kale, spinach, bell peppers, and other vegetables are great options because they are high in vitamins A, C, and K as well as important minerals like potassium and magnesium. By lowering oxidative stress and encouraging lung tissue regeneration, these nutrients support respiratory health.

Dinners that are appropriate for people with COPD must also include lean protein sources. Choose skinless chicken, fish (like salmon or mackerel) high in omega-3 fatty acids, and plant-based proteins (like tofu or lentils). Protein is essential for preserving muscle strength, particularly in the respiratory muscles, which can be weak in COPD patients.

When creating dinner meals, consider including whole grains as a rich source of complex carbs. Whole grains that provide a steady supply of fiber and energy, such as quinoa, brown rice, and oats, are beneficial for gut health. They also include important minerals including B vitamins, which promote energy production and a healthy metabolism.

Take into consideration employing herbs and spices that have anti-inflammatory qualities when seasoning your meal recipes. In addition to adding taste to your food, turmeric, ginger, garlic, and rosemary help to lower respiratory system inflammation.

Try a variety of cooking techniques to get the most nutrition out of your supper meals. Sautéing, baking, steaming, or grilling with little to no oil are all fantastic options. These techniques minimize the inclusion of extra lipids that can worsen respiratory symptoms while preserving the inherent flavors of the foods.

These meal recipes, which emphasize nutrient-dense and anti-inflammatory foods, are meant to please your palate while simultaneously promoting better respiratory health.

Some Advice for Making Appetizing and COPD-Friendly Dinners

Making delectable dinners that are COPD-friendly requires careful consideration of portion sizes, conscientious cooking methods, and carefully chosen ingredients. Start by organizing your meals such that they feature a range of foods high in nutrients and are specifically designed to meet the needs of people with COPD.

One important component of dinners that are COPD-friendly is portion control. Meals that are smaller and more frequent can be easier on the stomach and help people with respiratory issues avoid experiencing the uncomfortable sensation of being full. By dividing your meal into smaller servings throughout the day, you can make sure that your body is getting enough important nutrients without overtaxing your respiratory system.

For optimal nutritional intake and to sustain energy levels in between meals, choose nutrient-dense snacks. Nuts, fresh fruit, and raw veggies are good sources of vitamins, minerals, and antioxidants that can be obtained as snacks without adding unnecessary calories to your diet.

A healthy respiratory system depends on enough hydration, so drink lots of water during supper. Herbal teas, broths, and water are all great options. Sugary and caffeinated drinks should be avoided as much as possible as they can cause dehydration.

To improve the enjoyment of your COPD-friendly dinners, try experimenting with different flavor profiles. Use citrus flavors, herbs, and spices to give your food more depth and variation without using a lot of salt or heavy sauces. Fresh herbs, such as basil, cilantro, and parsley, can improve the flavor of your food.

Keep an eye out for any food allergies or factors that can impact respiratory symptoms. Even if some foods could be advantageous, it's critical to recognize your sensitivity. If certain substances seem to make symptoms worse, think about substitutes or seek individualized guidance from a healthcare provider.

You can prepare dinners that are not only tasty and fulfilling but also customized to the requirements of people with COPD by using these suggestions.

Protein, Carb, and Fat Equilibrium for Optimal Nutrition

A well-balanced supper requires careful consideration of sources of protein, carbohydrates, and fat to ensure adequate nutrition for those with COPD. Maintaining muscular mass, promoting general respiratory health, and supplying sustained energy all depend on the proper balance of these macronutrients.

Make dinner meals that include lean protein sources first. Good options include fish, poultry, tofu, lentils, and low-fat dairy products. Essential amino acids included in these proteins are required for the upkeep and repair of muscles. Maintaining muscle strength is essential for COPD patients since the illness can damage the breathing muscles.

Add complex carbs for a consistent energy release. Brown rice, quinoa, and whole wheat pasta are good examples of whole grains. In addition to providing your body with energy, these carbohydrates support digestive health and are a good source of fiber, both of which are good for general health.

Incorporate heart-healthy fats into your dinner preparations to aid in the absorption of nutrients. Omega-3 fatty acid sources like flaxseeds and fatty fish (salmon, mackerel) are very advantageous. Due to their anti-inflammatory qualities, these fats may be beneficial for those with COPD who may have persistent respiratory irritation.

To balance macronutrients and avoid overeating, mindful portion control is essential. To assist control portion sizes and prevent overtaxing the digestive system, use smaller plates. Those with COPD who may have dyspnea during or after meals may potentially benefit from this strategy.

Try a variety of cooking techniques to make sure your meal retains its nutritional value. Excellent options that reduce the need for additional fats while maintaining the natural flavors of the ingredients include grilling, baking, and steaming. Pay attention to additional oils and choose, in moderation, heart-healthy oils like avocado or olive oil.

Dinner recipes that meet nutritional requirements and improve the general health of patients with COPD can be made by emphasizing the balanced integration of proteins, carbs, and fats.

CHAPTER SEVEN

HEALTHY COOKING PRACTICES FOR THE RESPIRATORY SYSTEM
The Best Cooking Techniques to Keep Nutrients Safe:

Selecting cooking techniques that retain the nutritional content of the ingredients is crucial when respiratory well-being is the main concern. In this sense, steaming is the clear winner. By heating food with steam, this gentle cooking method makes sure that the majority of its vitamins and minerals are retained.

A straightforward and efficient way for beginners is to place a steamer basket over a kettle of boiling water. Vegetables like broccoli or carrots should be placed in the basket, covered, and allowed to steam naturally. This technique maintains a desired texture, intensifies the flavors, and retains nutrients.

Poaching is another useful method, particularly for protein sources like chicken or fish. Cooking in a simmering liquid—usually broth or water—helps preserve the nutrients and moisture during the poaching process. Beginners might begin by adding seasoned fish fillets to a tasty broth, gently simmering, and cooking until the fish is done. The end product is a delicious dish that is high in nutrients and meets the dietary requirements of those with COPD.

The secret is to roast at lower temperatures if you like the substantial flavors of roasted items. To achieve the desired caramelization, roasting vegetables or lean meats at a moderate heat helps preserve their nutritious value. For beginners, a straightforward method is to preheat the oven, season the selected components with herbs and spices, and roast them until they turn golden brown. A delicious balance between maintaining nutrition and producing visually beautiful, savory food can be achieved with this strategy.

Advice on How to Reduce Respiratory Irritants While Preparing Food:

For those with COPD, respiratory health is critical, and it's important to be aware of potential irritants when preparing food. For beginners, choosing whole, fresh ingredients whenever feasible is a sensible first step. Foods that have been processed and packed may have preservatives and additives that irritate the respiratory system. Novices can better manage what goes into their meals by starting with natural foods.

Strong smells and allergens can be released during chopping and slicing, particularly when using strong items like garlic and onions. Novices can use a well-ventilated space or think about handling the chopping with kitchen appliances like a food processor to reduce respiratory irritation. This facilitates a more comfortable cooking experience by lowering direct exposure to harsh scents and airborne particles.

A useful suggestion for beginners is to select non-stick cookware. Cooking in non-stick cookware uses less oil, which reduces smoke and other possible irritants. It's best to use oils with higher smoke points, such as canola or olive oil when using them. This keeps the cooking process seamless and pleasurable while lowering the possibility of producing respiratory irritants.

Cooking Utensils and Devices that Simplify Meal Preparation:

Having the appropriate appliances and equipment in the kitchen can make cooking a lot easier, especially for those who have COPD. A kitchen scale is an excellent purchase for beginners looking for a quick and easy method. For nutritional balance, ingredients must be measured precisely. A scale offers accuracy, guaranteeing that portion sizes meet dietary guidelines.

Another useful piece of equipment for beginners is an immersion or portable blender. These small appliances make it simple to puree sauces and soups right in the pot, doing away with the need to move hot liquids to a conventional blender. This makes cooking safer by lowering the possibility of spills and burns in addition to saving time.

 Purchasing a high-quality knife with an ergonomic grip will help beginners do tasks like chopping and slicing more easily. Less effort is needed to use a sharp knife, which eases hand and wrist strain. Cutting boards with non-slip surfaces also make kitchens safer places to be.

Therefore, beginner cooks may prioritize respiratory wellness for COPD patients by using practical tools and gadgets, following suggestions to reduce respiratory irritants, and choosing the proper cooking methods. These detailed instructions guarantee a guided and pleasurable cooking experience, promoting maximum satisfaction for anyone looking to improve their general health with a diet that accommodates COPD.

CHAPTER EIGHT

COPD HYDRATION TECHNIQUES

Maintaining Hydration Is Essential for Respiratory Health:

For those suffering from Chronic Obstructive Pulmonary Disease (COPD), staying properly hydrated is crucial to maintaining their respiratory health. Dehydration can worsen symptoms and impair lung function, so people with COPD must prioritize their fluid intake. Sufficient moisture is necessary for the respiratory system to support the mucous membranes lining the airways in the best possible way. These membranes can effectively collect and evacuate mucus and irritants when well-hydrated, minimizing airway obstruction and lessening the strain on already-compromised lungs.

The increased effort required for breathing, which frequently results in fast and shallow breathing, is a common worry for persons who have COPD. These problems can be made worse by dehydration, which can produce thicker mucus and more dyspnea. Dehydration may also exacerbate weariness, which in turn can put an additional load on the respiratory muscles. Consequently, a fundamental component of managing COPD is developing a habit that involves drinking enough water regularly.

Innovative Methods to Increase the Amount of Fluids in Your Diet:

Maintaining adequate hydration doesn't have to be a difficult or boring chore. Adding extra fluids to your diet can be done in a variety of fun and creative ways, which will make the process pleasurable in addition to being healthy. Try experimenting with infused water as a way to add fruit slices (such as cucumber, lemon, or berries) to your water to make it taste better without using sugar- or caffeine-filled drinks. This enhances the flavor of the water and adds extra nutrients that are beneficial to general health.

Including foods high in hydration in your diet is another tactic. Foods high in water content, such as celery, cucumbers, and watermelon, can make a big difference in how much fluid you consume each day. Soups and broths are great choices since they are high in water content and provide nutrients in a form that is easy to digest. Herbal teas are a pleasant option that may be tailored to your tastes and served hot or cold. By taking advantage of these inventive options, staying hydrated may be enjoyable and interesting.

Selecting Drinks to Help Lung Function:

Drinking the correct beverages is important for people with COPD because some choices might aggravate respiratory symptoms or be very beneficial for lung health. Water is by far the most important and dependable choice. It has no calories, thins mucus, and maintains the proper lubrication of the respiratory system. Herbal teas can also help to ease breathing by calming the airways, especially if they contain herbs like ginger or peppermint.

However, it's best to restrict your use of alcoholic and caffeinated drinks. These may act as respiratory irritants and worsen the symptoms of COPD by contributing to dehydration. Selecting non-alcoholic and non-caffeinated options, like diluted fruit juices or decaffeinated herbal teas, guarantees a more lung-friendly beverage selection. One proactive step in promoting normal lung function and general respiratory health is making educated beverage selections.

CHAPTER NINE

DEVELOPING MEAL PLANS ADAPTED TO COPD
Detailed instructions for creating customized food plans

When designing customized meal plans for people with COPD, it's important to take into account their dietary requirements and overall health objectives. Assessing the person's present eating habits, health, and any particular advice from medical providers is the initial stage in this procedure. It is essential to comprehend the individual's baseline nutritional intake and preferences to properly customize the meal plan.

Start by determining the essential nutritional elements that are critical to the management of COPD. These include consuming enough protein to maintain healthy muscles and eating meals high in vitamins and minerals and healthy fats to maintain energy levels.

Designing meals that are not only nutrient-dense but also pleasant is crucial, given the possible obstacles like decreased appetite and trouble chewing or swallowing.

Next, group foods according to the nutrients they contain. Give lean proteins (fish, poultry, and lentils) priority because they are high in necessary amino acids and low in saturated fats. To guarantee a wide range of vitamins and minerals, including a selection of vibrant fruits and vegetables. Add in whole grains, like brown rice and quinoa, for a longer-lasting energy boost.

Another crucial component of customized meal planning is portion control. Because appetite and energy expenditure might fluctuate in people with COPD, it's critical to adjust portion sizes to suit their unique requirements.

Since they are easier to digest and offer a consistent supply of nutrients, smaller, more frequent meals throughout the day may be advantageous.

It is equally crucial to take fluid intake into account. Dehydration may be more common in people with COPD, therefore it's important to encourage them to drink enough water throughout the day. Limiting alcohol and caffeine, two substances that might cause dehydration is also recommended.

Include the person in the decision-making process to increase the meal plan's practicality. Ask about their favorite meals, flavors, and textures to make sure the meal plan suits their palates. Remember to provide any dietary requirements or allergies so that the plan can be adjusted appropriately.

It is essential to monitor and modify the meal plan regularly. Periodic evaluation guarantees that the meal plan is efficient and flexible, even when an individual's health status and nutritional requirements may change over time. Working together with medical specialists, such as nutritionists or dietitians, can offer insightful advice at every stage of the procedure.

Lasting Meals throughout the Day to Provide Long-Lasting Energy

One of the most important tactics for treating COPD and encouraging sustained energy levels is to space out meals throughout the day. Instead of following the conventional three-meals-a-day schedule, start by distributing your consumption of food among a few smaller meals and snacks. This offers a steady supply of energy in addition to assisting with potential appetite swings.

A balanced breakfast that consists of a variety of carbohydrates, proteins, and healthy fats is a great way to start the day. Fruits, yogurt, and whole-grain cereals can all be great options. Including a dose of protein, like eggs or lean meats, aids with blood sugar stabilization and provides energy for the duration of the morning.

Choose nutrient-dense foods like nuts, seeds, or fresh fruit for mid-morning and afternoon snacks. These snacks supply important vitamins and minerals and give you a rapid energy boost without raising your blood sugar.

A balance of veggies, nutritious grains, and lean proteins should be the main focus of lunch and dinner. To create a visually pleasing and delightful dinner, use a range of colors and textures. A well-balanced plate includes grilled chicken or fish, quinoa or brown rice, and a big helping of vibrant veggies.

To balance meals for long-term energy, timing is essential. To keep your nutritional intake steady, try eating every three to four hours. Steer clear of big, heavy meals right before bed to avoid indigestion and discomfort. Encourage people to practice mindful eating by teaching them to pay attention to their bodies' signals of hunger and fullness.

Although it's sometimes forgotten, staying hydrated is essential for maintaining energy levels. Make sure you drink enough water throughout the day because being dehydrated can make you feel tired. Drinking infused water and herbal teas can vary your fluid consumption without adding any calories.

Modifying Meal Planning By Dietary Requirements And Personal Preferences

For long-term adherence and enjoyment, meal plans must be modified to accommodate individual preferences and dietary limitations. Assessing the person's culinary preferences, cultural background, and any dietary limitations they may have should be your first step. This data serves as the basis for developing a customized and entertaining meal plan.

To make the meal plan more enticing, include your favorite foods and flavors. Find inventive methods to incorporate a person's favorite ingredients or cuisine, provided that it maintains the nutritional balance required for COPD management. This improves the flavor of the food and encourages a positive outlook on dietary adjustments.

When creating the meal plan, consider any dietary restrictions, such as intolerances or allergies. It's essential to stay away from certain allergies and troublesome foods to avoid negative reactions. Collaborate closely with the person to find appropriate substitutes that satisfy their dietary requirements without sacrificing variety or flavor.

Meal planning should be flexible enough to accommodate individual preferences. Understand that there is no one-size-fits-all solution and that everyone has various likes and preferences. Permit personalization within the suggested dietary restrictions, giving the person the freedom to select foods that suit their preferences.

To accommodate a range of tastes, introduce variations in cooking techniques and textures. While some people might favor cooked vegetables, others might prefer the crunch of raw ones. Try varying the herbs and seasonings to bring out the flavors without using too much sugar or salt.

Encourage a slow switchover to the modified meal plan. Abrupt and significant changes could be too much to handle, which could result in resistance and even non-compliance. Gradually increase the extent of tiny alterations at first until the person feels more at ease with the new food regimen.

To facilitate adaptation, regular communication and feedback are essential. Regularly check in with the person to find out how they are feeling about the meal plan, resolve any issues, and make any necessary adjustments. The meal plan will always be a dynamic and changing tool that can be adjusted to meet the needs and preferences of the individual thanks to this collaborative approach.

CHAPTER TEN

EASY MEAL PREPARATION KITCHEN TRICKS
Time-saving advice for effectively preparing meals:

Even for people on a COPD diet, meal preparation can be time-consuming, but with a few ingenious tips, you can speed it up and make it more doable. Always start by organizing your meals for the upcoming week. This saves time and reduces the number of trips you need to make to the store by enabling you to shop for goods all at once and help you prepare a well-balanced diet.

Your prep time can be greatly reduced by setting aside time at the beginning of the week to chop vegetables and portion ingredients. Think about setting aside a particular day to chop and arrange ingredients. Put them in portion-sized containers so you can quickly get what you need each week without having to spend a lot of effort preparing ahead of time.

Choose recipes that have similar ingredients or flavors as well. In this manner, you can make bigger quantities of a base ingredient that you can use in several different recipes all week long. For example, make a big pot of brown rice or quinoa and use it as a side dish or in stir-fries and salads.

Take advantage of the appliances in your kitchen. Purchasing appliances such as a food processor, blender, or mandolin slicer can greatly expedite the process of dicing and slicing.

For people with COPD, these technologies not only save time but also make cooking more pleasurable and less taxing.

Finally, think about cooking with a friend or your family. This not only makes the procedure more pleasurable but also enables work division, which improves the efficiency of meal preparation.

Even beginners can learn the art of effective meal planning while sticking to a COPD-friendly diet by using these time-saving suggestions.

For Convenience, Prepare Meals In Bulk And Freeze Them:

For those on a COPD diet, batch cooking is revolutionary since it offers a practical means of always having wholesome, home-cooked meals on hand. Start by selecting a day of the week, preferably on the weekend, when you have a little more time to commit to batch cooking. This will reduce the amount of cooking you have to do each day by enabling you to prepare a stash of meals that can be quickly reheated throughout the week.

Make sure the recipes you choose can be frozen and cooked in bulk. Soups, stews, casseroles, and chili are great options because their flavors tend to get better over a couple of days in the refrigerator. These kinds of meals can be frozen for later use after being portioned into separate containers. To keep freshness and monitor expiration, make sure your containers are freezer-friendly and appropriately labeled with the preparation date.

To get the most out of your batch cooking efforts, double or triple the recipe while making meals. This lowers the frequency of cooking sessions while also saving time. It's simple to thaw and reheat precisely what you need for each meal when you portion the meals into serving sizes that meet your dietary requirements.

One way to facilitate the thawing process is to divide larger portions into single meals. In this manner, you can remove only the necessary amount without needing to defrost the entire batch. To avoid freezer burn and keep the quality of your food, use freezer-safe bags or containers and remove as much air as you can.

If you make bulk cooking and freezing a regular part of your routine, you'll soon have a freezer full of tasty, low-effort meals that are perfect for people with COPD every day. This method guarantees simplicity while also assisting you in keeping a steady, well-balanced diet.

Setting up your kitchen to make cooking easier for those with COPD:

A smoother and more enjoyable cooking experience can be greatly enhanced by creating an orderly and COPD-friendly kitchen. Sort through the items in your kitchen first. Clear out extraneous stuff from cupboards, drawers, and countertops to make your kitchen space hygienic and easily accessible. This lessens visual distractions and facilitates finding and reaching necessary objects.

Organize your kitchenware in a way that will reduce physical strain. To prevent unnecessary bending or stretching, keep commonly used things at waist level or close at hand. To make the most of your storage space and keep things within reach without requiring heavy lifting, think about investing in pull-out shelves or organizers.

Make sure your fridge and pantry are stocked with COPD-friendly meal options. Sort related items together to facilitate finding what you're looking for.

To guarantee that perishables are utilized before they expire and to prevent forgetting about them, keep them in the refrigerator at eye level.

It can also be quite beneficial to label shelves and containers, especially for others who might help in the kitchen. Confusion and potential accidents during meal preparation are decreased when items and utensils are clearly labeled, making it simple for everyone to identify them.

Invest in cooking appliances and tools that are COPD-friendly. For those with COPD, cooking might be easier using lightweight cookware and utensils with ergonomic designs. To lessen strain and manual labor, think about utilizing electronic appliances like food processors, blenders, and can openers.

By putting these organizing tips into practice, you can make your kitchen a COPD-friendly area that encourages effectiveness, use, and accessibility.

As a result, even individuals who are not experienced in the kitchen may cook with assurance and create meals that fit the COPD diet.

CHAPTER ELEVEN

EATING OUT WHILE HAVING COPD

Looking for options that are respiratory-friendly on restaurant menus:

When dining out, people with COPD need to choose their menu carefully because some foods can make their symptoms worse. When looking at the menu at a restaurant, choose dishes that are low in sodium because eating too much salt might make you retain fluids and make breathing harder. Lean protein options, such as grilled chicken or fish, are less prone to upset the stomach and are easy on the digestive tract.

A COPD-friendly diet should include plenty of vegetables, but it's important to stay away from ones that are high in chemicals that cause gas. Select cooked or steamed veggies over raw ones because the process of cooking breaks down potentially difficult-to-digest fibers. Leafy greens, like kale or spinach, are great options because they are high in vitamins and don't cause bloating.

Choose whole grains such as brown rice or quinoa for your carbohydrates because they are high in fiber and provide you energy for a longer period. Steer clear of oily and fried foods as they might cause respiratory irritation and inflammation. Rather, choose baked, grilled, or roasted menu items, as these cooking techniques lower the total fat level.

In addition, take into account portion sizes to avoid overindulging, which can overwork the respiratory system. Requesting a reduced portion or sharing a dish can be a sensible tactic. To make sure your selections are in line with your respiratory-friendly diet, don't be afraid to question your server about particular components or preparation techniques.

Notifying Restaurant Employees About Dietary Requirements:

When dining out with COPD, it's important to let the staff know exactly what you require in terms of dietary restrictions. Be precise and explicit about your preferences and limitations right away. Tell your server about any special needs you may have, such as dietary restrictions or a preference for prepared veggies.

A lot of eateries are accommodative and will change menu items to accommodate special dietary needs. To effectively manage your sodium intake, politely ask for adjustments, such as sauces or dressings on the side. Proactively communicate any allergies or sensitivities, stressing the value of carefully planning your diet.

Ask the chef to make a special dish for you if there are no options on the menu that meet your dietary requirements. The majority of establishments are accommodating, particularly if doing so guarantees their customers a satisfying dining experience.

Asking inquiries about the components in a particular cuisine, the cooking techniques utilized, and any possible substitutes is another important part of effective communication. It is more probable that the restaurant staff will collaborate with you to design a dish that fits your COPD-friendly diet when there is clear communication between you and them.

Techniques for keeping a diet that is COPD-friendly when dining out:

Efficiently adhering to a COPD-friendly diet when dining out requires implementing particular tactics that enable you to make knowledgeable decisions. Start by looking up and choosing eateries that have a reputation for serving healthier menu items. Nowadays, a lot of places offer nutritional data online, so you may schedule your meal ahead of time.

Eating smaller, more frequent meals throughout the day is another useful tactic that might assist avoid overindulging when dining out. If at all possible, eat a little snack before you leave the house to stave off impulsive, unhealthy restaurant decisions.

To help you make healthier choices, think about asking your dining partners for their support. Talk to them about your dietary preferences, and suggest going to eateries that offer a range of alternatives that meet your COPD-friendly standards. Eating out can be less stressful and more fun when you have a supportive network.

Furthermore, pay attention to portion sizes and your body's signals of hunger and fullness. If the restaurant offers bigger servings, think about splitting the dinner with a friend or getting a box to go with the leftovers. In this manner, you can enjoy eating out without sacrificing a diet that is COPD-friendly.

Finally, drink water throughout the meal to stay hydrated. For those with COPD, staying well hydrated is crucial because it supports the maintenance of optimum respiratory function. Reducing alcohol and sugar-filled drinks is advised because they can cause dehydration and may not be in line with a diet that is good for the respiratory system. By putting these tactics into practice, you may prioritize your COPD nutritional needs and dine out with confidence.

CHAPTER TWELVE

OVERCOMING CHALLENGES ASSOCIATED WITH COPD

Managing Typical Obstacles in Keeping a Healthy Diet When Living with COPD:

Chronic obstructive pulmonary disease, or COPD, comes with several difficulties that might make eating a balanced diet seem impossible. Nonetheless, people with COPD can overcome these obstacles and enhance their general well-being with the appropriate strategy. One of the most prevalent problems is managing weight since COPD can cause unintentional weight gain or loss. This highlights the requirement for a diet that balances regulating calorie consumption with supplying enough nutrients.

Changing the diet to meet the higher energy expenditure linked to laborious breathing is an important factor to take into account.

Foods high in nutrients become vital for making sure people with COPD get the vitamins and minerals they need without consuming too many calories. This balance can be attained by including whole grains, lean proteins, and a range of fruits and vegetables.

Managing dyspnea is another difficulty and can make eating an arduous and time-consuming activity. Smaller, more frequent meals spread throughout the day might help combat this.

In addition to keeping energy levels stable, this facilitates digestion via the respiratory system. Furthermore, concentrating on foods that are simple to chew and swallow can lessen the weariness that comes with eating.

The possible combination of some drugs with food is a serious concern. People with COPD must speak with their doctor about any dietary advice or limitations depending on their prescribed treatment plan. By taking a customized approach, it is ensured that the diet supports the medical treatment plan and helps manage overall health.

Techniques for Getting Past Obstacles in the Way of Meal Planning and Preparation:

For those with COPD, organizing and preparing meals can be very difficult, but with the correct techniques, these issues can be overcome. Starting with easy meals that can be prepared quickly and with little effort is a sensible first step for beginners. Choosing meals that need little preparation and cooking time will help you feel less exhausted and handle the cooking process better.

Making a menu in advance is a crucial tactic. This entails putting together a weekly or monthly food plan that accommodates both dietary needs and tastes. By dividing the plan into more manageable parts, people can stay organized and experience less stress when making daily meal decisions. Making use of meal plans to inform grocery lists expedites the shopping process and guarantees that essential components are constantly available.

Investing in kitchen appliances that simplify duties can be a game-changer for individuals who struggle with mobility.

Meal preparation may be made a lot easier with the help of appliances like pre-chopped veggies, a high-quality blender for smoothies, or a slow cooker for quick one-pot dinners. These gadgets make cooking more accessible by reducing physical strain and saving time.

Involving caregivers or family members in meal preparation might offer much-needed assistance. In addition to reducing the strain on the COPD sufferer, collaborative cooking promotes a sense of belonging and shared accountability. To further ensure that there are always wholesome, ready-to-eat options available and lessen the need for regular preparation, think about batch cooking and freezing portions.

Advice for Handling Nutritional Modifications and Adjustments:

Managing dietary modifications and alterations is an essential part of living with COPD. Starting small and making modest tweaks and adjustments is crucial to making this process easier for beginners. Making drastic dietary changes might be daunting; therefore, it is advisable to start modestly and adjust gradually.

Paying attention to hydration is a sensible first step. People with COPD must drink enough of water because it thins mucus and makes breathing easier. Consuming foods high in water, such as fruits and vegetables, can help maintain proper hydration. Getting into the habit of drinking water every day—especially during meals—is a straightforward yet powerful way to maintain respiratory health.

Healthcare providers may suggest nutritional supplements to make sure people with COPD get enough nutrients. Protein drinks, vitamins, and minerals are a few examples of these supplements. Beginners must follow their healthcare provider's recommendations on the right timing and dosage for these supplements and include them in their daily routine.

Another piece of advice for handling dietary changes is to keep a close eye on portion sizes. Meals that are smaller and more frequent can assist you in avoiding overindulging and using less energy during digestion. This strategy helps to sustain energy levels without overtaxing the respiratory system.

It can be advantageous to practice mindful eating as well. A better relationship with food can be achieved by chewing food fully, taking the time to enjoy each bite, and paying attention to signals of hunger and fullness. This enhances general well-being in addition to the dietary component.

In summary, managing obstacles to eating a balanced diet when living with COPD necessitates a multimodal strategy. People with COPD can improve their quality of life and better manage their illness by adopting practical meal preparation procedures, knowing the unique dietary demands, and making doable dietary alterations.

CHAPTER THIRTEEN

MAINTAINING A LIFESTYLE COMPLIANT WITH COPD

Long-term methods for implementing a diet suitable for people with COPD in daily life:

Adopting a COPD-friendly diet entails long-term methods that can dramatically enhance the quality of life. Living with COPD requires a careful approach to nutrition. Priority one should be given to eating a well-balanced diet that consists of a range of foods high in nutrients. This comprises entire grains, fruits, vegetables, lean proteins like fish and chicken, and healthy fats. A varied and nutrient-dense meal that offers vital vitamins and minerals to support general health might be indicated by a colorful plate.

Another essential component of a diet suitable for people with COPD is knowing how to regulate portions. Meals should be smaller and more often throughout the day because overeating can cause pain and put greater strain on the respiratory system. This method not only facilitates better digestion but also helps control energy levels, avoiding the exhaustion that sometimes follows heavier meals.

For those suffering from COPD, staying hydrated is crucial as it facilitates breathing and thins mucus. A COPD-friendly lifestyle revolves around consuming enough water, and adding herbal teas and low-sodium broths can help with overall hydration. Alcoholic and caffeinated drinks should be avoided as they might cause dehydration.

A useful tactic to make sure a COPD-friendly diet becomes a regular part of life is meal planning. It is possible to better control nutritional intake and prevent impulsive, potentially hazardous food choices by taking the time to prepare meals and snacks in advance. Furthermore helpful is maintaining a food journal, which offers insights into eating habits and permits modifications as necessary.

Recognizing Accomplishments And Making Necessary Corrections:

Starting a COPD-friendly diet requires being flexible and appreciative of little accomplishments. Acknowledging successes promotes a good outlook, whether they have to do with managing weight, having more energy, or improving general well-being. Sustained achievement requires this kind of encouragement.

The secret to enjoying achievements is to set reasonable and attainable goals. Divide more ambitious goals into more doable, smaller tasks to enable a methodical approach that inspires confidence and drive. Smaller modifications like increasing the amount of fruits and vegetables in each meal or sticking to a regular exercise schedule improve general health.

Making changes to your lifestyle to make it more COPD-friendly is inevitable. Being adaptable is essential since people's wants and situations might change.

If dietary preferences or constraints change, be willing to adjust the meal plan as necessary. Consultations with healthcare providers regularly might yield insightful information and direction for making wise decisions.

Motivation And Support To Help People With COPD Live A Healthy Lifestyle:

With COPD, maintaining a healthy lifestyle demands constant inspiration and support. It's critical to have a network of friends, family, and other COPD patients around oneself for support. A sense of community is developed from sharing struggles and experiences, and the encouragement from one another can be quite motivating.

A crucial component of maintaining motivation is incorporating fun physical activities into the schedule. Engaging in activities that correspond with one's interests and physical capabilities increases the appeal of exercising. This can involve exercises like swimming, walking, or even mild yoga.

Enhancing endurance and respiratory function can be achieved by progressively increasing the duration and intensity of these exercises.

Deep breathing exercises and meditation are examples of mindfulness activities that improve mental and physical health. These techniques can aid in the management of stress and anxiety, two conditions that people with COPD frequently face. Maintaining a healthy lifestyle is mostly dependent on having a good mindset, and practicing mindfulness can be a useful tool in this regard.

Consultations with medical professionals regularly offer chances for continued support and inspiration. A supportive environment is established for people managing COPD through progress tracking, problem-solving sessions, and individualized guidance. Honoring accomplishments, no matter how minor strengthens the will to lead a healthy lifestyle and motivates ongoing work toward achieving optimal well-being.

In summary

Key Ideas For A Diet Suitable For People With COPD Are Summarized:

Before starting the path to improved respiratory health through diet, it is important to review the fundamentals of what makes a diet suitable for people with COPD. These guidelines are intended to improve the general well-being of those suffering from Chronic Obstructive Pulmonary Disease (COPD) in addition to relieving symptoms.

First and foremost, it's critical to keep the right ratio of nutrients. To effectively treat the symptoms of COPD, a diet high in lean proteins, healthy fats, complex carbs, vitamins, and minerals is recommended. Proteins are essential for maintaining and repairing muscles, especially in those with COPD who may develop muscular atrophy. Because of their anti-inflammatory qualities, essential fats like omega-3 fatty acids can help reduce respiratory system inflammation.

Simultaneously, complex carbohydrates—found in whole grains and vegetables—offer a steady supply of energy without quickly elevating blood sugar levels. Those with COPD who may feel exhausted and breathless can especially benefit from this. A balanced diet rich in vitamins and minerals, particularly antioxidant-rich ones like vitamins C and E, boosts immunity and fights oxidative stress, which is a typical issue with COPD.

Hydration also has a major influence. Patients with COPD frequently struggle with dehydration, which can make symptoms worse. Drinking enough water makes mucus thinner, which makes breathing easier. Striking a balance is crucial, though, as consuming too much fluids can put strain on the heart. Monitoring fluid consumption regularly is advised.

Another essential component of a diet that is COPD-friendly is portion control. Eating more often and in smaller portions can help the respiratory system work less hard during digestion. This method also aids in weight management, since being overweight exacerbates the symptoms of COPD.

It's also important to stay away from specific food triggers. Processed foods with a lot of sodium can cause water retention, which puts more strain on the heart and lungs. While moderate consumption of alcohol and caffeine may be appropriate for certain people, it's important to keep an eye on them as they might exacerbate dehydration.

MY GRATITUDES

Dear Valued Readers and Supporters,

I hope this message finds you well. I am writing to express my deepest gratitude to both God and each one of you for the overwhelming support and positive response to my book. Your encouragement and enthusiasm have truly touched my heart, and I am immensely thankful for the journey we are on together.

I believe that every success is a result of collaboration and support from various sources. First and foremost, I want to acknowledge the divine guidance and inspiration that led me to create this cookbook. Without the grace of God, this endeavor would not have been possible.

To my cherished readers, your commitment to exploring healthier dietary options for managing your crises has been both inspiring and humbling. Your trust in this book" means the world to me, and I am honored to be part of your journey toward improved health and well-being.

Also, I am reaching out to kindly request your valuable feedback on this book. Your thoughts and insights are crucial in helping me enhance and serve you better, ensuring that it continues to meet your needs effectively. Please take a moment to share your thoughts by rating and writing reviews on platforms where the book is available.

Your reviews not only provide me with invaluable feedback but also play a significant role in assisting others in making informed choices. By sharing your experiences, you contribute to a community that values health and wellness, creating a positive impact on countless lives.

Additionally, I encourage you to share this book with your friends, family and loved ones. Together, we can extend the reach of this promising resource, offering support and guidance to those who may benefit from it. Having this knowledge and seeking medical advice from your specialist I anticipate a turnaround for us.

Once again, thank you from the depths of my heart for your unwavering support. I am committed to continually improving and serving you better. Let us continue this journey together, promoting health, well-being, and a shared sense of community.

With sincere appreciation,

[Emmy Brooks]

Author, "COPD DIET COOKBOOK"